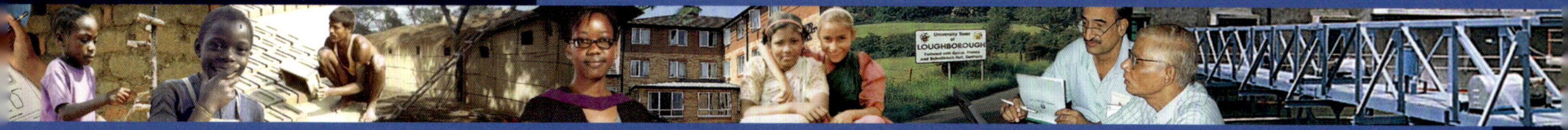

Comparing National Sanitation Policy Content

An initial review of nine country profiles

Summary

As part of research assessing the effectiveness of national sanitation policies, in 2003 the contents of 9 national policy documents were reviewed:

- Bangladesh – National Policy for Water Supply and Sanitation, 1998
- Cambodia – National Policy on Urban Sanitation, September 1999
- Ghana – Environmental Sanitation Policy, published 1999
- Indonesia – National Policy for the Development of Community-Managed Water Supply and Environmental Sanitation Facilities and Services, 2002 (draft 3)
- Mozambique – National Water Policy, 1995
- Nepal – National Sanitation Policy, July 1994
- Nigeria – National Water Supply and Sanitation Policy, 2000
- South Africa – White Paper on Basic Household Sanitation, 2001
- Uganda – National Environmental Health Policy for Uganda, April 2003 (draft)

The review addressed questions concerning key elements of policy, as identified in the USAID's Environmental Health Project (EHP) report Guidelines for the assessment of national sanitation policies (Elledge et al, 2002, Section 3). Additional questions provide background information on the scope of the policy, when and how it was produced.

Findings of this review are in the table that follows.

Key findings

- **Targets and resources**: None of the policies attempt to quantify targets or identify the resources to be budgeted for sanitation improvements other than in a very general way.
- **Assessment of the existing situation**: Few of the policies provide more than a very general assessment of the existing situation in the country to which they relate. Some reflect the current thinking and priorities of international agencies.
- **Targeted groups**: Some, but not all, policies make reference to the specific needs of target groups, e.g. the urban poor, residents of small towns, inhabitants of rural communities. In most cases, reference is made to the needs of some of these groups. A few make very general reference to programmes or budgets targeted at these groups.
  - The Uganda policy makes reference to the needs of urban and peri-urban populations, while the South Africa policy focuses on the needs of rural communities and informal settlements.
- **Minimum levels of service**: None of the policies specify minimum service levels, although broad reference is given in the South Africa policy.
- **Related ministries**: In most cases, neither the Ministry of Health nor the Ministry of Environment has been specifically mentioned as being involved in the preparation of policy.
  - In South Africa, both ministries were represented in the Task Team that developed the policy. In Uganda the Ministry of Health is the lead agency.
- **Health considerations**: Most of the policies reviewed have a specific concern with health.
  - The South Africa and Uganda policies provide background information on the types and magnitude of health problems arising from poor sanitation.

Loughborough University

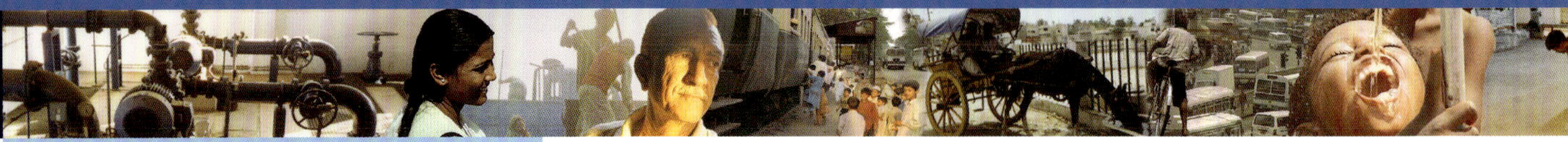

Sanitation finds a home in South Africa

Lack of sound institutional frameworks is a major cause of failed sanitation provision. Sanitation rarely has a clear institutional "home", resulting in fragmented responsibilities, lack of ownership and poor coordination.

South Africa has pioneered "joined-up thinking" through its innovative national sanitation policy; a particularly striking feature is the multi-sectoral approach to sanitation provision. Whilst overall responsibility for sanitation rests with a specific department, the programme development and implementation is actually achieved by multi-sectoral partnership involving the household, local government, NGOs, private sector, provincial government and the central government. The institutional and organizational framework clearly defines the roles and responsibilities of these stakeholders[1].

- **Environmental considerations**: Most policies include general references to the need to protect the environment, but none indicates the magnitude of sanitation-related environmental problems.

- **Cost of sanitation**: Few of the policies provide any indication of the cost of meeting sanitation needs.

  - The South Africa policy provides information on the maximum capital and O&M cost per household.

- **Subsidies for capital**: Most policies allow for some subsidy of capital costs.

  - The Ghana policy explicitly allows financial allocations from national government to subsidize the recurrent costs of municipal systems. The Uganda policy states that capital subsidy should be allowed for the poorest, those living in areas with poor ground conditions, tenants and people in transit.

- **Hygiene education**: The Nepal, South Africa and Uganda policies refer to the need to fund hygiene education. However, only South Africa defines what the subsidy should be (R600 per household at the time) and identifies its source (Department of Water Affairs and Forestry).

- **Institutional arrangements**: Most policies provide general rather than specific guidance on institutional policies and roles. Some provide general guidance on the options for correcting institutional weaknesses. Most, but not all, policies identify a lead agency for coordinating sanitation activities.

  - The South Africa policy is the only one to clearly identify roles and responsibilities for related government ministries (Ministry of Health, Education).

- **Technical/social aspects**: Most policies recognize the need to take account of concerns relating to both technical ('hardware', such as design options for latrines) and social ('software', such as awareness raising) aspects of sanitation provision. Some give a good balance between these concerns, while others focus mainly on software aspects of provision.

  While social aspects may dominate in the wording of policy; allocation of budgets, roles and responsibilities, together with specific aspects relating to hygiene education, are not clearly identified. The concern for social aspects may therefore be more theoretical, responding to perceptions of current best practice, rather than enabling action at the community or household level.

Questions	Bangladesh	Cambodia[1]	Ghana	Indonesia	Mozambique	Nepal	Nigeria	South Africa	Uganda
General questions									
Is the policy separate or combined with water supply?	Combined	Separate	Separate	Combined	Combined (called national water policy)	Separate – with guidelines for planning and implementation	Combined	Separate	Separate – within Environmental Health policy
What is the scope of the policy (urban/rural, comprehensive/ poverty focused)?	Comprehensive (urban/rural)	Urban	Comprehensive (urban/rural)	Community-based services	Comprehensive (urban/rural)	Comprehensive (urban/rural)	Comprehensive (urban/rural)	Focuses on rural and informal settlements	Comprehensive (urban/rural)
When was the policy prepared?	1998	1999	1999	2002	1995	1994	2000	2001	2003 (review ongoing 11/03)
Who prepared the policy?	Government department[2]	Consultant	Government	Consultant?	Government Department?[3]	Government department[4]	Consultant?	Government – National Sanitation Task Team	Government – Ministry of Health
What provision was made for consultation on the policy?	Not clear but probably limited	Discussions with 48 focus groups, govt officials etc.	'Extensive' consultation	Consultative process to produce policy	Not identified	Not identified	Not clear but probably limited	Consultation within the Task Team, involving range of Government Ministries	Not identified
Legal framework (Section 3.3)[2]									
Are roles and responsibilities clear and appropriately assigned to institutions?								Yes	No
Has the policy been formally adopted? (Question in Guidelines is whether the existing legal framework adequately covers sanitation)	Yes	No	Yes	Approved by deputy minister	Not clear (probably yes)	Yes	No	Yes	No - policy currently in review process (Nov '03)

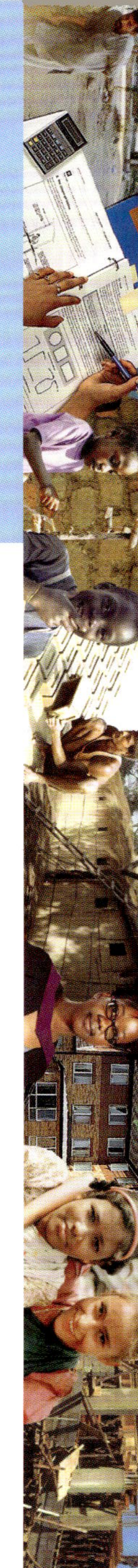

Questions	Bangladesh	Cambodia[1]	Ghana	Indonesia	Mozambique	Nepal	Nigeria	South Africa	Uganda
Outputs & targets (Section 3.4)									
Does the policy refer to specific outputs and targets? (Note: this and the following four questions are not included in the Guidelines, but have been added as they seem relevant).	Yes	Yes	Yes	Yes (in a rather general way)	Yes	Objectives are general, but refer to targets of HMGN[5]	No (targets for water supply clearly stated)	Yes - State President's Office target of basic minimum level to all by 2010	No - objectives and aims are given in general terms
Are targets quantified where appropriate?	No	No	Generally no[6]	No	Yes (specifically for urban areas)	No	No (except for water supply)	No	No
Are institutional targets included?	Yes	Yes (responsibility for sanitation management	Yes	Yes	No	No	No	No	No
Does the policy indicate a time-frame for the achievement of targets?	No	No	No	Refers to 5yr implementation period	Yes (by end of 2000)	No	No	Yes - by 2010	No
Does the policy relate the targets to the existing situation and current problems	No	No (relates more to recent WSP thinking)	No	No (relates more to international agency priorities	Yes	No	Yes	Yes - states number of h/h without access to sanitation	N/A
Does the policy make specific reference to the needs of rural communities, small towns and poor urban communities?	Rural and urban communities considered separately	Urban groups - which implicitly include poor communities	No	Yes - in so far as focused on small community-based schemes	Not specifically	Identifies need for separate rural/urban plans, etc. Priority to most densely populated urban/semi-urban areas	Yes, especially rural communities	Policy focuses on rural communities and informal settlements. Priority to communities without basic level of service, with greatest health risk	Yes - mentions problems for urban and peri-urban population in the introduction
Does the policy make reference to either programmes or budgets for the targeted groups	No	No	No	Only in a very general way	Yes	No	No	No	Considers funds for schools, health units, refugees, low income h/hs, & geographically difficult areas

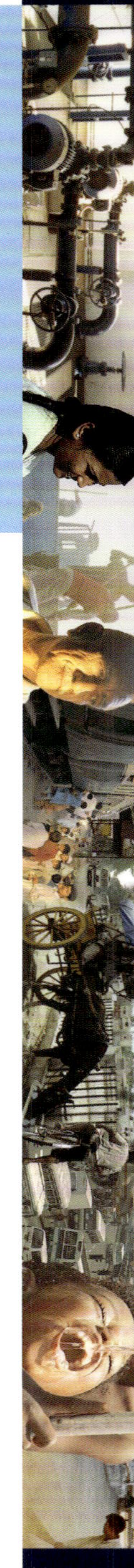

Questions	Bangladesh	Cambodia[1]	Ghana	Indonesia	Mozambique	Nepal	Nigeria	South Africa	Uganda
Levels of service (Section 3.5)									
Does the policy define minimum service levels for the targeted population groups	No	No (but reference to technology choices)	No	No	No	No	No	Broadly: hygiene awareness & behaviour, disposal systems, toilet facility per h/h	No
Are these service levels appropriate in the light of existing and planned water supply services	N/A	N/A	N/A	N/A	N/A	N/A	N/A	N/A	N/A
Health considerations (Section 3.6)									
Did the Ministry of Health play a role in national policy formulation?	No	Not clear but probably not	Minor role at most	No	No	Not identified	Not clear - probably not	Yes, part of Task Team	Yes - lead agency
Is health an explicit concern of the policy?	Yes	Passing reference – main focus on sanitation as economic and social good	No	Yes (but main aims relate to quality of life)	No	Yes - within definition of sanitation, statement, directive and objectives	No	Yes - within definition, problem statement and principles	Health is of primary concern
Does the policy provide information on the types and magnitude of the health problems arising from poor sanitation?	No	No	Types to some extent	No	No	Identifies IMR[7] in the introduction	No	Yes, with incidence of diarrhoea in children <5yrs	Yes
Does the policy address these health problems?	N/A	N/A	To some extent	N/A	No	Yes - in directives and objectives	No	Yes, with hygiene behaviours	Yes - primary aim and vision

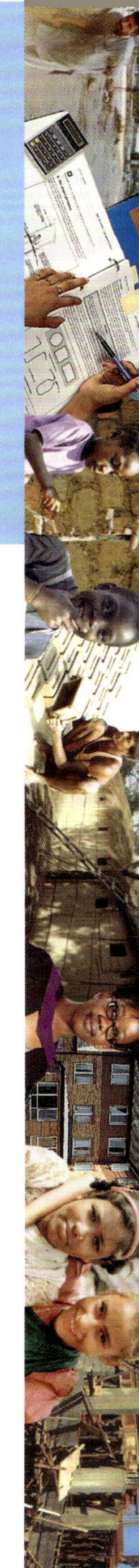

Questions	Bangladesh	Cambodia[1]	Ghana	Indonesia	Mozambique	Nepal	Nigeria	South Africa	Uganda
Environmental consideration (Section 3.7)									
Did the Ministry of Environment play a role in national policy formulation?	No	Not clear but probably not	Minor role at most	No	No	Not identified	No	Yes, within Task Team	Not identified
Does the policy make specific reference to the protection of the environment	Yes	Yes, but as with health rather in passing	Yes (but rather in passing)	General references	No	Yes - in the introduction, in the definition of sanitation and the policy statement	No	Yes, in problem statement, definition and principles	Yes - in some detail
Does the policy provide any indication of the magnitude of sanitation-related environmental problems?	No	No	No	No	No	No	No	No	Not specifically - only in general terms
Does the policy address the main environmental problems?	Not explicitly	In a very general and perhaps not realistic way	In a very general way	General reference to raising community environmental awareness	N/A	Reference made to specific problems in legislation - but no details	Not really	Yes, through integrated environment planning, education and adopting a 'polluter pays' approach	Yes, throughout
Financial considerations (Section 3.8)									
Does the policy indicate the cost of meeting sanitation needs (capital, recurrent or both)?	No	No	No	No	No	No. States no programme will be 100% subsidised. Beneficiary contribution according to socio-economic status	No	Both - capital and O&M cost per household (max.) given	No, but identifies percentage of work-time lost due to sanitation-related sickness and injury
Does the policy indicate how those costs might be met?	N/A	N/A	N/A	N/A	N/A	Not in detail - independent budget for sanitaiton from national budget	N/A	Yes - identifies sources of funding: Equitable Share, grants, & revenue	N/A

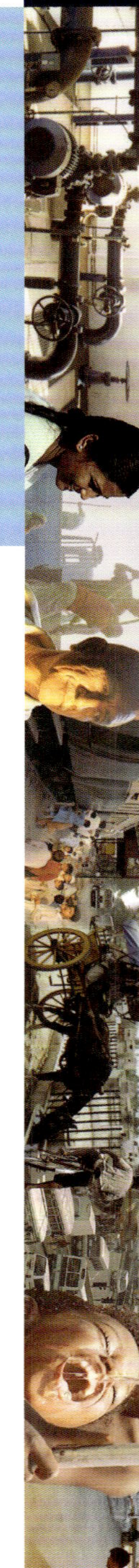

Questions	Bangladesh	Cambodia[1]	Ghana	Indonesia	Mozambique	Nepal	Nigeria	South Africa	Uganda
Does the strategy for meeting costs include subsidies on capital costs?	Not covered	For zonal and 'city-wide' facilities	Where necessary	N/A	N/A	Yes - but states not 100%	Yes (individual families are soley responsible)	Yes - one-off subsidy per h/h for community development (R600) and infrastructure (R600)	Only for specific conditions - poorest, poor ground conditions, tenants & people in transit
Does the policy assume financial allocations from national government to subsidize recurrent costs for municipal systems?	Not covered	No (explicitly requires that customers bear recurrent costs)	Yes (because sanitation high % of DC expenditure)	No - focus on self reliant local management	Not stated but implied	Not identified	Not covered	Available via the Equitable Share, together with tariffs set for water services	Encourages NGOs/CBOs - on cost-recovery basis
Does the policy refer to the need to fund hygiene education and other programmatic costs?	No	No - appears to assume demand exists	Only for HRD and operational research	No	No	Yes	No	Yes - with R600 subsidy per h/h	Yes
If so, are sources of funding identified and are they likely to be adequate	N/A	N/A	Not explicitaly identified	N/A	N/A	Not explicitly - identifies min. 20% of budget to be allocated to software aspects	N/A	Financed by Dept. of Water Affairs and Forestry (DWAF)	Not identified
Institutional roles and responsibilities (Section 3.9)									
Does the policy define institutional roles relating to planning, financing, regulation, implementation, O&M, M&E and programme support?	Some roles defined but in fairly general terms	Broad division between community and govt responsibilities	Yes (but need to check 'buy-in' by stakeholders)	Only in very general sense that govt is seen as facilitator of community action	No	Yes in general. More details in accompanying Guidelines for Planning and Implementation	In very broad terms - focused more on water supply	Yes - for municipal, provincial and national government, private sector and NGOs	Yes - from h/h to national government, but not in a clearly structured way
Does it provide guidance on correcting any institutional weaknesses?	No	No	Some reference to developing human resources	No	N/A	Some reference to restructuring and co-ordination committee to be formed	No	Through support from private sector & NGOs, co-ordinaiton groups and Sanitation Directorate within DWAF	Yes - with strategies to implement policy - setting up Board, training, co-ordination and communication

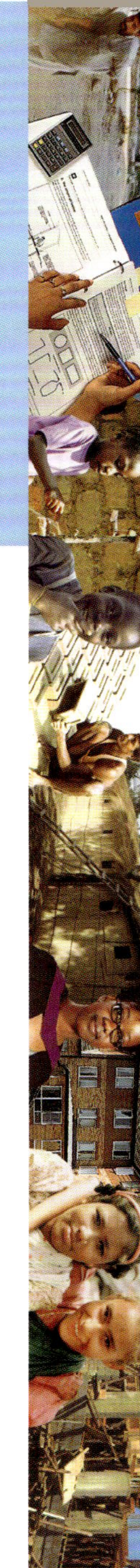

Questions	Bangladesh	Cambodia[1]	Ghana	Indonesia	Mozambique	Nepal	Nigeria	South Africa	Uganda
Does it identify a lead agency for co-ordinating sanitation activites?	No	No	Yes - Ministry of Local Government and Rural Development (MLGRD)	No	No	Yes - MoHPP[8]	No	Yes - DWAF	Yes - Mistry of Health Environmental Health Division with plan to establish Environmental Health Board
General (Section 3.10)									
Does the policy recognize both technical (hardware) and social (software) concerns?	Yes	Yes	Yes	Yes	Yes	Yes	Yes	Yes	Yes
Which of the two predominates?[9]	Reasonably balanced	Reasonably balanced	Reasonably balanced	Software	Hardware	Software	Hardware	Software	Software

Notes

Information relating to the policy context, legislation and other supporting procedures is based only on information found in the policy document itself.

(1) Analysis based on executive summary
(2) Local Government Division – Ministry of Local Government and Cooperatives
(3) National Directorate of Water
(4) Environmental Sanitation Section (ESS) of the Department of Water Supply and Sanitation (DWSS), within the Ministry of Housing and Physical Planning (MoHPP) – the lead agency
(5) His Majesty's Government of Nepal - targets of "Health for All 2000" and "Basic Minimum Needs"
(6) There is a target of 100% sanitation coverage, by either domestic toilets or hygienic public toilets.
(7) Infant Mortality Rate
(8) Ministry of Housing and Physical Planning (now the Ministry of Physical Planning and Works (MPPW))
(9) This question is not easy to answer. Most policies make considerable reference to software aspects of policy but their intention is to ensure that the hardware is provided.

Note that the following issues are not explicitly addressed: Gender, monitoring and evaluation, poverty, water quality monitoring, private sector, promotion and awareness raising, schools and other institutions, aligning policy with other sectors – such as education, women's development, water resources, etc.

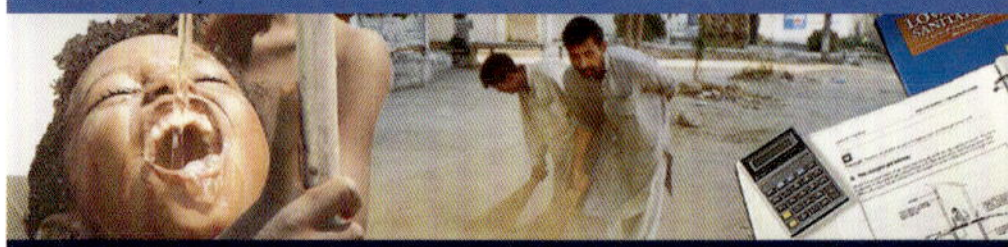

This Briefing Note presents a comparison of key elements of national sanitation policies, based on a desk-review of the content of nine country policies carried out in 2003.

It is based on the findings of research undertaken in 2003-2005, as part of a DFID-funded research project *Application of tools to support national sanitation policies* (R8163).

Other research outputs include:

- Sanitation Policy: Why it is important and how to make it work – an overview guidance note
- National sanitation policy in Ghana: a case for improved co-ordination? – a briefing note from Ghana
- Implementing national sanitation policy in Nepal: challenges and opportunities – a briefing note from Nepal

Key references

Elledge, M. F., Rosensweig, F. and Warner, D. B. (2002). *Guidelines for the assessment of national sanitation policies* (EHP strategic report no.2), Arlington, USA. Available at http://www.ehproject.org/PDF/Strategic_papers/SRSanPolFinal.pdf (accessed Sept 05).

Published by WEDC, November 2005

This Briefing Note is part of a series covered by ISBN 1 84380 093 4 and was funded by the UK Department for International Development (DFID). The views expressed, however, are not necessarily those of DFID.

WEDC *People-centred solutions for sustainable development since 1971*

For more information contact:

Rebecca Scott or Andrew Cotton
Water, Engineering and Development Centre (WEDC)
Department of Civil and Building Engineering
Loughborough University
Leicestershire LE11 3TU UK

Telephone: +44 (0) 1509 222885
Fax: +44 (0) 1509 211079
Email: r.e.scott@Lboro.ac.uk
a.p.cotton@Lboro.ac.uk
Website: http://wedc.Lboro.ac.uk/projects/new_projects3.php?id=142

Footnotes

1 WEDC *Application of Tools to support national sanitation policies* Inception Report for DFID KaR Project R8163 (unpublished), WEDC, 2003.

2 Section numbers refer to corresponding sections in the EHP Guidelines.

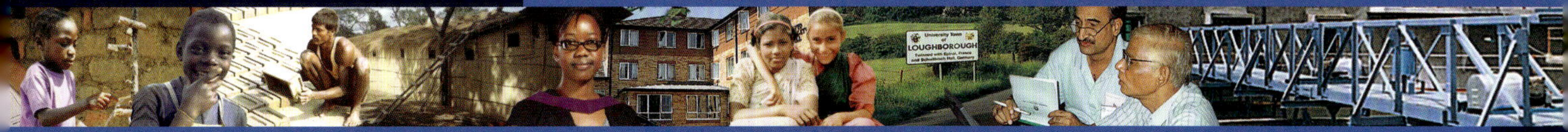

Sanitation Policy

Why it is important and how to make it work

WEDC

Summary

This note is concerned with sanitation policy, what it is, why it is important and what can be done to ensure that it is relevant and can be effectively implemented. It draws directly on research work carried out in Nepal and Ghana and indirectly on experience from several other countries.

Improved sanitation can contribute both directly and indirectly to the Millennium Development Goals, but this contribution is unlikely to be achieved in the absence of appropriate sanitation policies – which help to provide the overall framework within which change and improvement can take place.

Sanitation policy is more likely to have an impact if it stands alone rather than forming part of a combined water and sanitation policy. However, policy can only make a difference if governments want it and are prepared to implement it.

With this in mind, this note provides guidance on generating support for policy improvements and ensuring that policy leads to action.

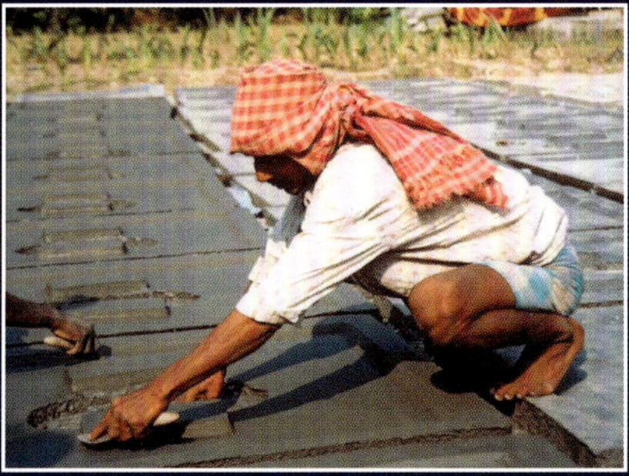

Headline findings

- Policy is important. It provides the framework within which improved sanitation services can move from isolated projects to national programmes. It is an important tool for the achievement of the MDG sanitation target[1].
- Policy documents should be concerned with overall objectives, the principles to follow and institutional roles and responsibilities to achieve those objectives. A strategy/action plan, plus guidance materials, can support a short policy document.
- Policy recommendations must not be implemented unless they are realistic, based on a sound assessment of existing conditions, problems and opportunities and accounting for the resources needed and available.
  - Policy targets for sanitation coverage in Nepal and Ghana are unrealistic, given the insufficient resources allocated to achieve these targets. Policy makers do not always account for what is already happening in the field.
- The policy development process can be used to generate interest and support in sanitation and improved sanitation policy.
- To be effective, policies must be widely owned. Those leading the policy development process must be able to engage with a wide range of stakeholders, to convince them of the value of policy.
  - Policies are often formulated at departmental level, with limited follow-up to ensure that senior decision-makers in affected ministries and organizations are committed to their implementation.
- Policy must link to PRSPs[2] and other national drivers of change.
- There is a need for greater focus on implementing policy and learning from experience.
  - NGOs that are active in the sanitation sector, such as Nepal Water for Health (NEWAH) in Nepal and WaterAid in Ghana, should be fully engaged in the policy development process.

Loughborough University

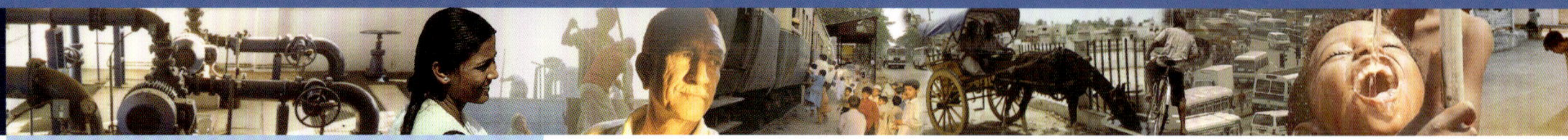

Sanitation and the Millennium Development Goals

The international community is committed to achieving the Millennium Development Goals (MDGs) and their associated targets.

- Reductions in the worm infections and diarrhoea resulting from improved sanitation and hygiene will help to increase people's productivity and so contribute to Goal 1, 'Eradicate extreme poverty and hunger'.
- The convenience, security, health and education benefits resulting from improved sanitation are likely to accrue particularly for women and will thus contribute to Goal 3 'Promote gender equality and empower women'.
- Target 5, to 'reduce by two thirds, between 1990 and 2015, the under-five mortality rate', is dependent on action to provide hygienic sanitation facilities and deliver effective hygiene education.
- Target 10, to 'halve by 2015 the proportion of people without sustainable access to safe drinking water and basic sanitation', is explicitly concerned with sanitation. Improved sanitation will also contribute to the achievement of other goals.
- Target 11, to 'achieve a significant improvement in the lives of at least 100 million slum dwellers by 2020', requires action to provide improved sanitation in slums.

Halving the proportion of people without access to improved sanitation will not be easy. Sanitation provision has historically lagged behind that of other services and few governments invest as much in sanitation provision as they do in drinking water facilities. Examples opposite show that current rates of sanitation provision in Nepal and Ghana will have to be increased if the target is to be achieved. It will then be important to ensure that sanitation facilities are used. Good policy, grounded in existing realities and widely recognized and supported can contribute to the achievement of these objectives.

Policy – what it is and why it is important

Policy is *'the set of procedures, rules and allocation mechanisms that provide the basis for programmes and services'* (Elledge et al, 2002). It is normally set out in a written document and must be supported by suitable policy instruments. These include laws and regulations, economic incentives, such as subsidies and fines for unsafe waste disposal, and information and education programmes, designed to create demand for improved sanitation services.

Policy provides the framework within which those who are seeking to improve sanitation can operate. A bad policy may constrain efforts to introduce effective sanitation services. For instance, a policy that states that municipalities must provide piped sewerage may prevent the development of more appropriate forms of sanitation in low-income and low-density areas. Conversely, good policy can:

- provide a clear focus for action by setting clear objectives and targets;
- ensure that stakeholder organizations are clear about their roles and responsibilities and what they can expect from others[4]; and
- ensure that there is general agreement on the principles and practices to be followed, for instance in relation to subsidies.

Why sanitation and hygiene need their own policy

In many countries, sanitation is considered along with water supply in a national water and sanitation policy. In others, the policy covers solid waste disposal in addition to excreta disposal and drainage. A combined policy can take account of the strong links between water, sanitation and health. Unfortunately, the institutional requirements of water supply and sanitation may be very different, particularly where most sanitation facilities are 'on-plot'.

Most combined policies focus on water supply and deal with sanitation in a rather perfunctory way. For instance, Nepal's Rural Water Supply and Sanitation Policy focuses strongly on community management but has little to say about the role of individual households, which are likely to have a major role in sanitation provision and management. If sanitation is to be given due attention, it needs its own policy.

Guidelines for the assessment of national sanitation policy

There is a clear need for guidance on the development, assessment and improvement of sanitation policy. The 'Guidelines for the Assessment of National Sanitation Policies' (Elledge, et al, 2002), identify *a process* that starts with the collection of background information and moves on to more detailed consideration of 'key elements' required to ensure successful policy formulation and implementation.

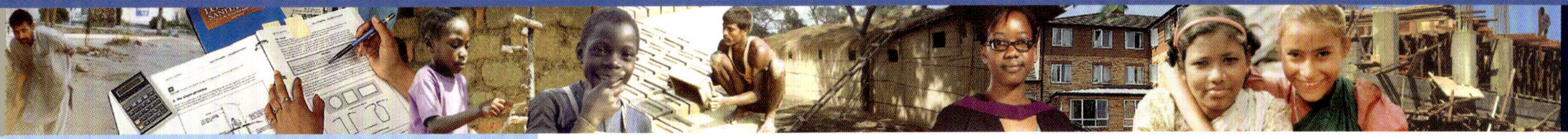

The challenge – achieving increased coverage and use

In Nepal, WaterAid (2004) estimate that sanitation coverage rose from 18% in 1990 to 27% in 2000. Expansion of coverage will have to be significantly increased if there is to be any chance of halving the proportion of people with access to improved sanitation by 2015.

Approximate estimates suggest that the total sanitation investment required to meet the MDG goals in Ghana will be of the order of $1 billion, of which around 75% will be for urban facilities. At the current rate of investment, rural sanitation coverage may actually fall from a current figure of around 31% to about 24% in 2015[3].

Policy content

The Ghana policy and the various Nepal policies all contain an overall target for sanitation coverage. These targets are probably too ambitious. More detailed targets are normally best left to back-up documents, such as strategies and action plans.

Ghana's policy which sets out the problems and issues to be addressed, explains the role of sanitation in achieving wider development goals, identifies overall objectives, states principles and identifies, in broad terms, the roles and responsibilities of the various stakeholders.

This note provides additional information to help place the Guidelines within the wider policy development process. It is based on workshops and consultations with key stakeholders in Nepal and Ghana, held over a 12 month period of the research.

Presenting policy – lessons from Nepal and Ghana

Nepal has developed a conceptually attractive method of presenting policy. A short policy document is associated with one or more back-up documents that provide additional information to support the implementation of policy. The 1994 National Sanitation Policy is supported by Guidelines. A more recent combined rural water and sanitation policy (2004) is supported by Strategies and Sectoral Strategic Action Plan.

When following this approach, it is important to be clear about the purpose of the various documents. The role of the Policy itself should be to establish overall goals, specify broad roles and responsibilities and identify key principles.

The strategy should provide more information on the approach to achieving the overall goals, identifying intermediate objectives and specifying who will be responsible for achieving them. It might include information on action to be taken to develop support for policy, the role of government financed programmes in supporting policy and the use of pilot and demonstration projects as an aid to achieving policy, together with more detailed guidance on roles and responsibilities.

The role of Action Plans is to set out the short- to medium-term actions required to implement the strategy while that of Guidelines is to provide additional information on implementation. To be useful, documents have to be reasonably detailed. Nepal has recently developed national Guidelines for Sanitation and Hygiene Promotion, 2005 to support the 1994 National Sanitation Policy. It would perhaps be more appropriate to produce a number of guidelines on specific topics, rather than trying to produce one Guidelines document to cover every aspect of sanitation.

What are the conditions for policy to make a difference?

Both Ghana and Nepal have serviceable, if not perfect, sanitation policies. Yet, both countries are some way from achieving their overall policy goals. The research suggests that it is not sufficient to look only at policy. Rather, it is necessary to also consider the conditions that need to be in place for policy to make a difference. These conditions relate to:

- *The context*. Are key stakeholders committed to improving sanitation facilities and implementing policy? If not, it is unlikely that any policy, no matter how good, will be implemented.
- *The policy itself – is it clear and realistic*? An unclear policy can be interpreted in different ways or ignored. A policy that is not grounded in a realistic assessment of existing conditions, problems and possibilities will

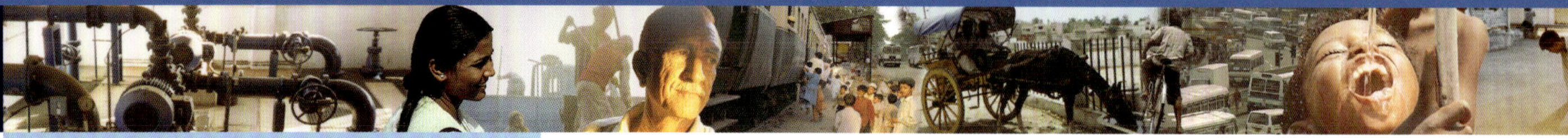

Key policy principles

Key policy principles include:

- The approach to be taken in relation to demand, subsidies and cost recovery.
- The approach to incentives, in particular the way in which incentives to communities as a whole might be used to support efforts to achieve 100% coverage.
- The need to support initiatives to improve sanitation services, wherever they occur, rather than tightly prescribing who can and cannot take such initiatives.
- The need to take a wide view of sanitation, encompassing hygiene behaviour and links with other services.
- The need for plans and programmes to take account of gender, vulnerable groups and environmental concerns.

The process chart shown here was used to develop and guide the policy assessment *process* in Nepal and Ghana.

It provides a development of the current process diagram for policy assessment, as provided in the EHP Guidelines.

The process chart can be used to decide where you need to start and what you need to do to introduce/improve sanitation policy.

Whilst the chart shows *generating support* and *developing policy* as separate activities, it is possible that the process of developing policy can be used to generate support for that policy and its prescriptions.

appear irrelevant to field workers. In both cases, the result will be that the policy has little or no impact.

- *Stakeholder awareness of the policy and its implications*. If those who are required to implement policy do not know about it, they cannot implement it. This implies a need to pay attention to the ways in which information on the policy and its implications can be disseminated.
- *Stakeholder acceptance of the policy*. Policies are unlikely to be widely accepted unless they are both clear and relevant. However, clarity and relevance are not enough. Policies must also be broadly owned, in the sense that stakeholders feel that the policy responds to their concerns, priorities and needs. We will see shortly that breadth of ownership is directly related to the process through which the policy is developed.
- *The quality and relevance of policy support instruments*, including amendments in legislation and procedures, strategies, action plans and programmes.

The policy development process

The starting point for policy improvement will depend on the existing situation and in particular the extent to which there is political will to review and produce/revise policy.

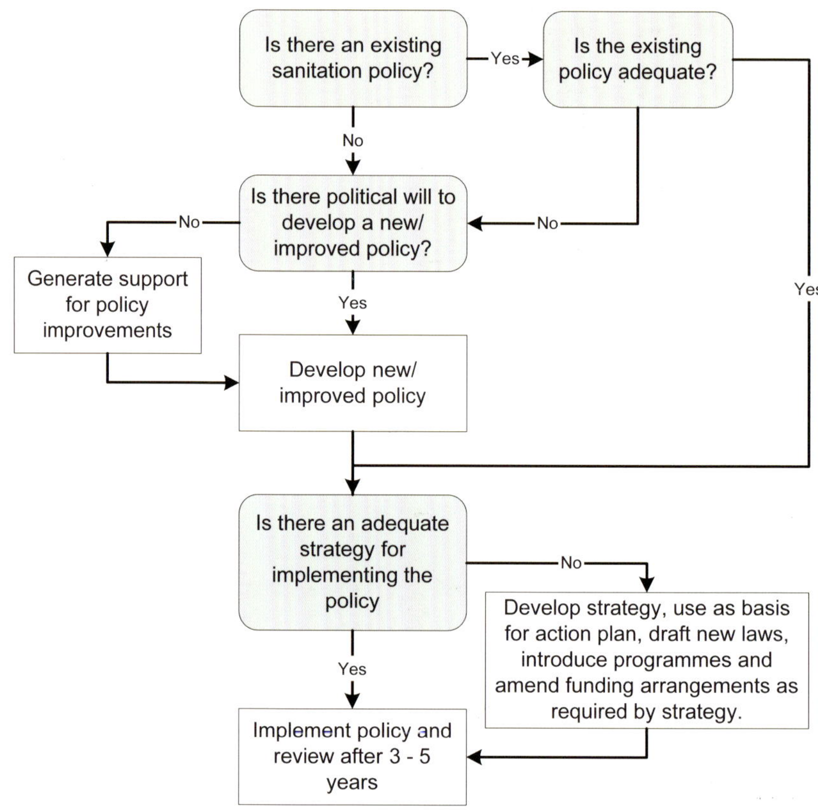

Figure 1. The policy development process

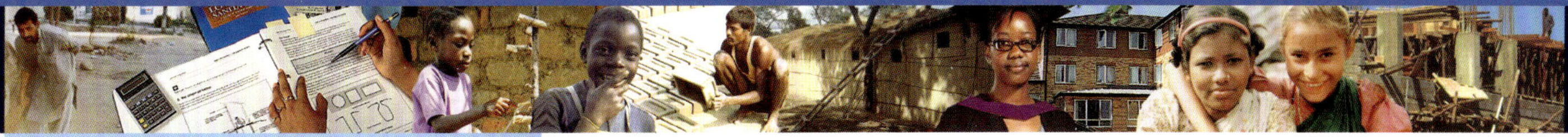

- In Ghana, most external funding is channelled through combined water and sanitation projects, which are implemented by the Community Water and Sanitation Agency (CWSA). CWSA is not even mentioned in Ghana's Environmental Sanitation Policy which appears to focus mainly on water supply.
- Nepal's Department of Water Supply and Sewerage does have a dedicated sanitation cell but this is small. Decentralization in Nepal has led to decisions on infrastructure priorities being made at the District level and below and institutions at these levels rarely prioritize sanitation. The 1994 sanitation policy in Nepal recognised the need to introduce sanitation-related expertise at these levels, but unfortunately its staffing recommendations were not implemented. A lack of specialist sanitation expertise at these levels of government means that the situation is unlikely to change.

The process used to develop the Rural Water Supply and Sanitation Policy in Nepal (under the Asian Development Bank's PPTA[5], 2002/2003) was overtly participatory. A wide range of stakeholders was involved in a series of workshops at which issues were identified and discussed and elements of policy were agreed. The consultants who led the process identified the following limitations in the process.

- It is relatively expensive and is therefore unlikely to be undertaken without donor support.
- Workshops can identify the areas in which consensus exists, but do not provide a good forum for resolving contentious issues.

Political will for policy improvement

In both Ghana and Nepal, the research suggested that sanitation currently has a low profile, as compared with water supply and other policy concerns. These findings point to the need to generate support for sanitation provision in general and for policy improvement and implementation in particular.

The policy assessment processes in the two case study countries suggest that a workshop can provide a good starting point for developing awareness of the need for change and that follow-up contacts and discussions, by either an individual consultant (Nepal) or a 'core' stakeholder group (Ghana), can further develop and spread awareness of the need for change. However, workshops are unlikely to attract the support of the high level politicians and officials, without which talk of policy improvement is unlikely to lead to action.

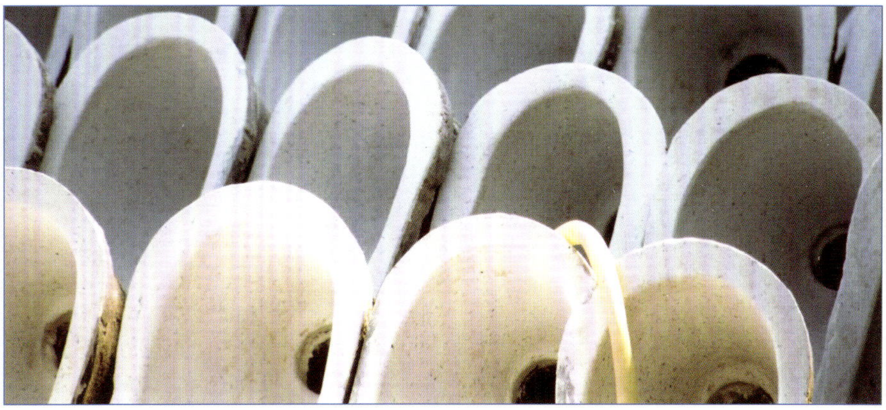

Developing new/improved policy

Where current policy is inadequate, assessment of policy should lead into the development of new improved policy. The research suggests that policy is normally formulated, and policy documents produced, by either a consultant or a team from the department that is leading the policy development process.

One key to the subsequent implementation of the policy is the extent to which those leading the policy development process are able to engage with a wide range of stakeholders and convince them of the value of the policy. Interviews with key stakeholders in the development of sanitation policy in Ghana and Nepal suggested that there was some such engagement in both countries but that this did not extend to all stakeholders and was insufficient to ensure that all aspects of policy were widely known and accepted.

A key point relating to both awareness-raising and policy formulation is the difficulty in ensuring that senior decision-makers from ministries and departments other than the lead ministry will attend workshops. This means that workshops cannot, in themselves, ensure that the policy is widely agreed and accepted **at the highest level**. This is particularly important where government systems are strongly hierarchical, so that most important decisions are made at the highest level.

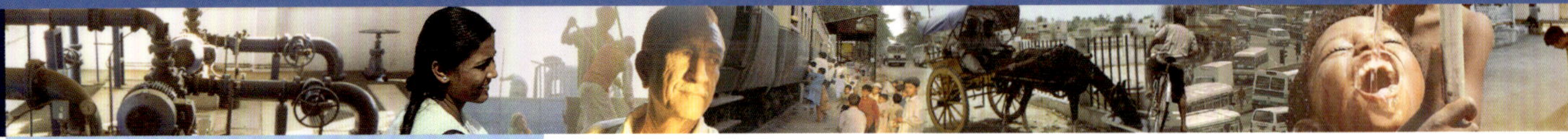

The experience of Ghana and Nepal suggests that relatively small amounts of donor support can help to establish and sustain high-level coordination bodies. It will normally be particularly important to draw representatives of national planning bodies and the Ministry of Finance into deliberations on policy and its importance. Indeed, coordinating bodies are most likely to be effective if they enjoy support at the highest level, most importantly from the national Planning Ministry.

Implementation of policy is more likely if the policy is linked to key government documents such as a country's Poverty Reduction Strategy Paper (PRSP) or equivalent. If sanitation is a central element in the PRSP, ministries and departments, from the Ministry of Finance down, together with donors, will be committed to providing resources for sanitation improvement. They will therefore be more likely to view sanitation policy as important. Sanitation is referred to briefly in the Approach Paper for Nepal's 10th Five Year Plan, which doubles as its PRSP. It is also mentioned in the Ghana Poverty Reduction Strategy. Here the problem may be the failure of the current sanitation policy to define a role for CWSA and the consequent tendency for CWSA and its donors to work outside policy.

The role of high-level coordination bodies

One response to the need for better inter-ministry, inter-departmental and inter-agency coordination is to form permanent high level working groups, coordinating bodies and steering committees. In addition to facilitating coordination, such bodies can also make the case for sanitation and facilitate the dissemination and implementation of sanitation policy. To function effectively, these bodies will often need financing and some form of secretariat, to ensure that their recommendations are acted upon.

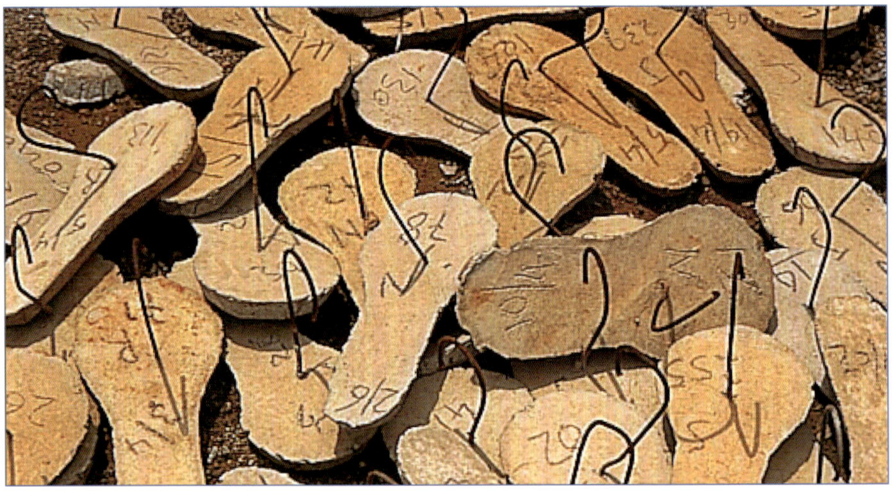

Adequate strategies for implementing the policy

The objective of a policy assessment and development process should never be solely to produce a policy. Rather, the aim should always be to ensure that the policy has a positive impact on national sanitation services. This requires systems and procedures to ensure that the policy is implemented. At the national level, this may require:

- enactment of new laws and sanctioning of new norms and procedures to support policy recommendations;
- an increase in the budget allocated to sanitation and hygiene promotion; and
- the implementation of plans and programmes to support the policy.

Local authorities can increase the budget that they allocate for sanitation in their areas but more general budget increases will require action by national government.

Overall, these findings suggest that policies must be realistic, must take account of all the stakeholders and be linked to PRSPs and other drivers of change. Remove any one of these conditions and policy is unlikely to be successful.

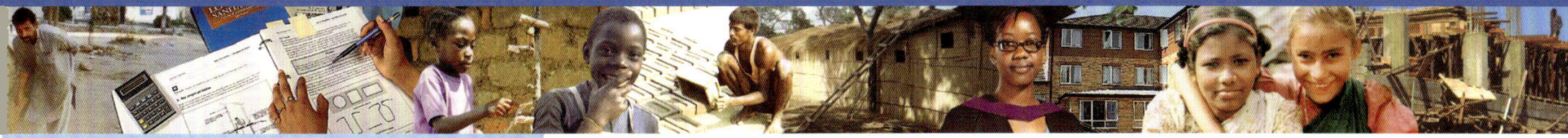

Key steps in assessing national sanitation policy

In summary, the key steps in assessing national sanitation policy, using the EHP Guidelines as a guide, are proposed as follows:

- Determine the best approach to carry out the assessment (refer to Section 1), ensuring that those leading the policy review process can influence subsequent implementation of that policy.
- Assess the current sanitation situation by obtaining realistic, relevant data (Section 2). Assess targets given in PRSPs, existing policy and other overarching documents to realistic targets, given the current situation and available/ required resources.
- In consultation with a broad group of stakeholders, determine the status regarding key elements of policy (Section 3).
- Analyse the findings and present these to the broad stakeholder group, providing opportunities for discussion, amendments, agreement and recommendations.
- Discuss and agree mechanisms for incorporating recommendations into policy review procedures.

The process chart in this note can be used to check the status regarding progress with amendments to policy, strategy and implementation procedures.

Linking the policy to drivers of change

The sanitation policy is more likely to be implemented if it is linked to the initiatives that are driving change in the country. In the first instance, it may be possible to link policy development to high-profile events. For instance, Nepal's Minister for Physical Planning and Works attended the South Asian Conference on Sanitation (SACoSan) in Dhaka in October 2003. However, it is not clear that this visit did lead to renewed efforts to implement or improve sanitation policy. This suggests that one-off events on their own are insufficient to bring lasting change.

Some key issues

Decentralization

Both Ghana and Nepal have gone through a process of decentralization and this is reflected in their sanitation policies. In both countries, the lead role in service provision is now assigned to local government entities, which fall under the local government ministry. In Ghana, the Ministry of Local Government and Rural Development (MLGRD) is also the ministry with responsibility for sanitation policy. However, even in Ghana, national and regional government entities are required to move from a providing to an enabling role. In practice, the capacity of local government in both countries is very limited and it appears that the specialist sanitation agencies continue to play a major role in service provision. So, there is a gap between what is prescribed by decentralization policy and what actually happens. Sanitation policy can respond to this situation by:

1. Explicitly considering the action to be taken to taken to create/strengthen local government sanitation-related capacity.
2. Clearly setting out the role to be played by specialist agencies, both in the short and the longer term. This role may at times involve rather more than facilitating the work of other organizations. When considering possible roles always follow the golden rule that 'policy prescriptions must be realistic'.

Capacity-building recommendations must clearly state whose capacity is to be built and for what purpose.

Subsidy

Sanitation policy must clearly state who should pay for sanitation services. Government should focus on promotion and higher order facilities, such as main sewers and treatment works, which protect the wider environment. Users should normally fund the construction of latrines and pay for their operation. Any subsidies for poor people should be clearly identified and explained. Even where significant subsidies on public facilities are allowed in the short term, the policy should say something about the desirability of reducing them over time.

Increasing the focus on sanitation

The research suggests that sanitation continues to be linked to water supply, often in the role of the 'junior partner'. In Nepal, a joint rural water supply and sanitation policy has recently been produced, despite the fact that there is already a sanitation policy. In Ghana, international agencies continue to channel funds through CWSA for joint water and sanitation programmes, which are heavily weighted towards water supply.

Evidence from other African countries, including Ethiopia and Tanzania, suggests that Ghana is not unique in this respect. There is a need for a much greater emphasis on sanitation in both policies and programmes. Given the very different institutional frameworks required for piped water supply and on-plot sanitation services, it will often be appropriate to develop specific sanitation programmes rather than seeing sanitation as an add-on to water supply.

Encouraging innovation

Policy should encourage innovative approaches to sanitation provision. Examples of such approaches from the case study countries include the introduction of school-led 'Total Sanitation' in Nepal and the involvement of small private sector artisans to support sanitation marketing and implementation in Ghana.

The aim should not be to specify how and where innovations should be attempted but rather to recognize their value and make provision for small amounts of funding where appropriate.

Footnotes

1 The Millennium Development Goal (MDG) sanitation target is to halve the proportion of people without improved sanitation by 2015.

2 Poverty Reduction Strategy Papers.

3 Based on figures contained in report prepared by Lukman Y. Salifu as part of a joint WEDC/WaterAid investigation of sanitation policy in Ghana.

4 Non-government organizations play an important role in sanitation provision and hygiene promotion in both Nepal and Ghana. Policy can facilitate the roles played by such organizations by recognizing their activities and clarifying their relationship to government systems.

5 Project Preparation Technical Assistance.

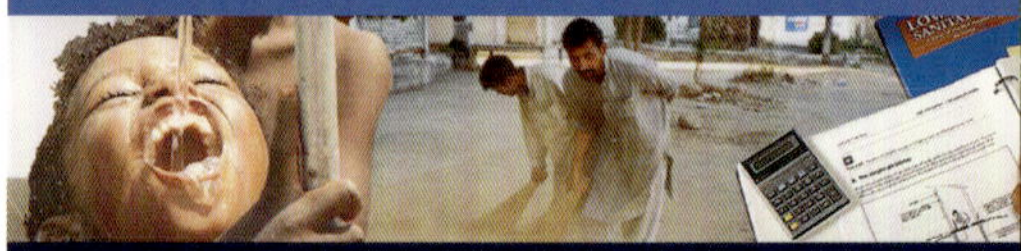

This Briefing Note presents key aspects of sanitation policy; what it is, why it is important and what can be done to ensure that it is relevant and can be implemented effectively.

It is based on the findings of research undertaken in 2003-2005, as part of a DFID-funded research project *Application of tools to support national sanitation policies (R8163)*.

Other research outputs include:

- National sanitation policy in Ghana: a case for improved co-ordination? – a briefing note from Ghana.
- Implementing national sanitation policy in Nepal: challenges and opportunities – a briefing note from Nepal.
- Comparing National Sanitation Policy Content – a note summarising and comparing the content of sanitation policies from 9 countries.

Key references

Elledge, M.F., Rosensweig, F. and Warner, D.B. (2002). *Guidelines for the assessment of national sanitation policies* (EHP strategic report; no. 2). Arlington, VA, USA. Available at http://www.ehproject.org/PDF/Strategic_papers/SRSanPolFinal.pdf (accessed Sept 2005).

WaterAid, Nepal (2004). *The Water and Sanitation Millennium Development Targets in Nepal: What do they mean? What will they cost? Can Nepal meet them?*, Available from WaterAid Nepal. Email: wateraid@wateraid.nepal.org.np

Information on the 2003 Ghana Poverty Reduction Strategy is available at http://siteresources.worldbank.org/GHANAEXTN/Resources/Ghana_PRSP.pdf (accessed Sept 2005).

The Nepal Government's 10th Plan, which doubles as its PRSP is available at http://siteresources.worldbank.org/NEPALEXTN/Resources/Nepal_PRSP.pdf (accessed Sept 2005).

This briefing note has been compiled by:
Kevin Tayler, independent consultant
Rebecca Scott, WEDC

Photographs by Rebecca Scott and Darren Saywell

Published by WEDC, November 2005

This Briefing Note is part of a series covered by ISBN 1 84380 093 4 and was funded by the UK Department for International Development (DFID). The views expressed, however, are not necessarily those of DFID.

WEDC *People-centred solutions for sustainable development since 1971*

For more information contact:

Rebecca Scott or Andrew Cotton
Water, Engineering and Development Centre (WEDC)
Department of Civil and Building Engineering
Loughborough University
Leicestershire LE11 3TU UK

Telephone: +44 (0) 1509 222885
Fax: +44 (0) 1509 211079
Email: r.e.scott@Lboro.ac.uk
a.p.cotton@Lboro.ac.uk
Website: http://wedc.Lboro.ac.uk/projects/new_projects3.php?id=142

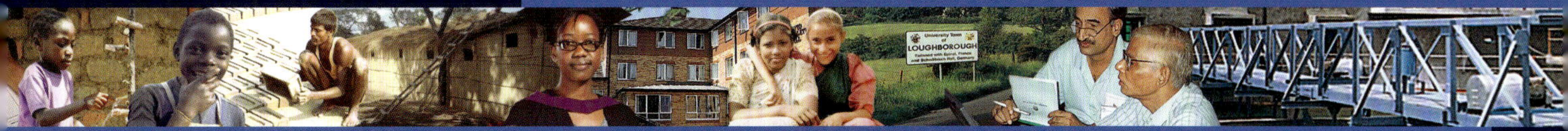

Implementing National Sanitation Policy in Nepal

Challenges and Opportunities

WEDC

Summary

Current national sanitation coverage in Nepal is reported to be in the range of 18-30%. There is an urgent need to meet the backlog and to cater for the sanitation needs of an increasing population.

Policy can set priorities, state principles and establish roles and responsibilities, so providing the framework within which these needs can be addressed. Nepal has had a national sanitation policy since 1994. While elements of the 1994 policy have been implemented, the situation is complicated by the existence of more recent rural and urban policies, covering both water and sanitation.

Overall policy objectives are framed in terms of the sanitation coverage to be achieved and the institutional arrangements for implementing policy. There is scope for improvements in the content of policy but the main issue in Nepal is how to effectively implement policy.

National Guidelines for Sanitation and Hygiene Promotion, 2005 are currently being developed, with the aim of strengthening the implementation of policy.

A significant increase in the rate of sanitation provision will be required to meet coverage objectives. This suggests a need to widen the number of organisations actively following policy and fulfilling the roles set for them by policy. In particular, increased engagement of the Ministry of Health could help to ensure effective sanitation promotion through the involvement of its community-based volunteers. Increased involvement of the National Planning Commission and the Ministry of Finance would help to ensure sanitation policy requirements are reflected in Nepal's poverty reduction strategy and 10 year plans.

Headline issues

- Despite the best efforts of government departments, international agencies and NGOs, over 70% of Nepal's population is still without access to safe sanitation.

- Estimates of sanitation coverage vary considerably but the available figures suggest that the current rate of increase in sanitation coverage is insufficient to meet the MDG sanitation target, let alone Nepal's stated policy objective of achieving 100% sanitation coverage by 2017.

- Nepal has had an approved national sanitation policy since 1994. A recent process to review the policy has resulted in the development of National Guidelines for Sanitation and Hygiene Promotion, 2005. Whilst intended to support implementation of earlier policy, the adoption of guidelines as opposed to a new policy document, suggests that not all stakeholders are convinced of the need for continual review and approval of separate sanitation-related policy.

- The National Guidelines for Hygiene and Sanitation Promotion, 2005 reflect Nepal's overall commitment to decentralization. While this aspect of policy is widely recognized by stakeholders, there are concerns about the lack of capacity in local government bodies to implement sanitation programmes.

- Implementation of policy is hampered by ongoing political and social instability.

Loughborough University

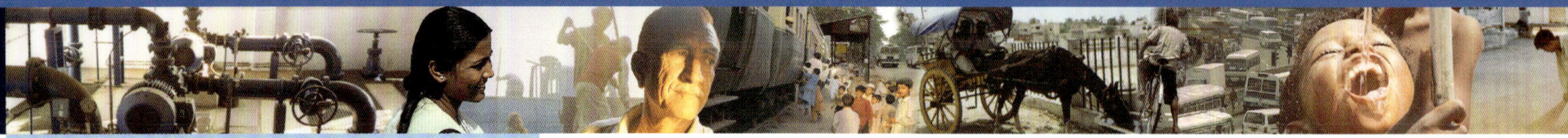

Background

Population

Nepal's population in 2001 was approximately 23 million, growing at a rate of about 2.25% per annum (national census of 2001). It is expected to reach over 30 million by 2015. At around 13% of overall population, the urban population is still fairly low compared with other South Asian countries. However projected figures suggest that the absolute growth in urban population to 2015 will almost match that in rural areas and will thereafter predominate.

Growth is significant in both smaller towns and the Kathmandu valley, with the Terai region (southern lowlands) experiencing higher urban growth than hill and mountain regions.

Health

Infant and under-five mortality rates remain high throughout Nepal. The Department of Health Services Annual Report for 2001/2002 reveals that, nationally, infection with intestinal worms, which is directly attributable to poor sanitation and hygiene, was over 7%, while overall morbidity levels associated with poor sanitation were rated at over 40% for all regions.

Sanitation coverage

Estimates of sanitation coverage vary widely. The commonly used coverage figures are 6% in 1990 and 25% in 2002[1]. A recent WaterAid report, consolidating estimates and drawing on the results of a number of assessments, suggests that national sanitation coverage increased from 18% in 1990 to 27% in 2000[2]. WaterAid notes that these figures are consistent with available information on levels of investment and per capita expenditure.

Efforts to expand sanitation coverage have been hampered by the ongoing internal conflict and instability, which makes access to many rural areas either difficult or impossible. Work continues in some districts, through the involvement of NGOs, who are able to reach rural areas that are closed to government officials.

Introduction

The Environmental Health Programme (EHP) of USAID developed Guidelines for the Assessment of National Sanitation Policies in 2002, to help countries assess sanitation policy in enabling an environment that encourages effective programmes and strategies. Nepal was selected as one of two countries for field-testing the relevance of the EHP Guidelines, as part of DFID-funded research carried out by WEDC in collaboration with Development Network, a national consulting and research firm in Nepal.

Using the EHP Guidelines as the basis for areas of policy assessment, a series of stakeholder workshops were held in Nepal during 2003 and 2004, supported by one-to-one consultation with individuals representing key national, regional and local-level institutions involved in sanitation. This provided opportunities to review and analyze both the content and, more importantly, the implementation of national sanitation policy – a key challenge facing Nepal as a whole.

Nepal's sanitation policy development

Nepal's first National Sanitation Policy was produced in 1994. The Policy itself is concise and is supported by a longer set of guidelines for planning and implementation contained in the same publication. An unofficial revised version, produced in 2002, was not ratified by the government.

The government approved a new National Rural Water Supply and Sanitation Policy, developed with Asian Development Bank technical assistance, in April 2004. This policy focuses strongly on rural water supply and does not consider sanitation in the same detail as the 1994 sanitation policy. The main policy document is again kept short and contained in the same document as a supporting Strategy. Additional information is provided by a separate 'Strategic Action Plan'.

Two further initiatives began more recently:

- Following a process to review the 1994 National Sanitation Policy, the lead government Ministry and Department have opted for the outcome of the review to be development of new National Guidelines for Sanitation and Hygiene Promotion, 2005. While clearly linked to the 1994 policy, these guidelines are a substantially new document – focusing on the implementation of policy, within the context of ongoing decentralization and the more recent Rural Water Supply and Sanitation Policy 2004.

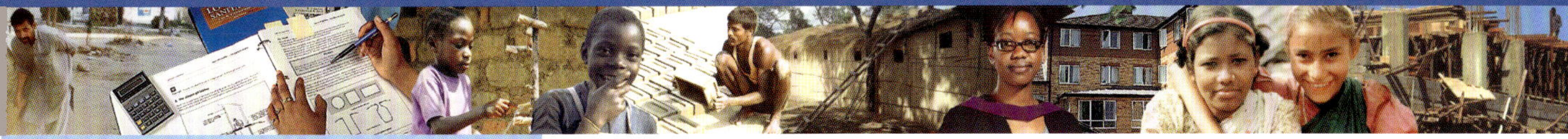

- The development of a National Urban Water Supply and Sanitation Policy in 2004. Policy development is being supported by the Japan International Cooperation Agency (JICA). Like the National Rural Water Supply and Sanitation Policy, the main focus of this document is on water supply. At the time of writing, this policy document is in draft format.

Institutional context

In common with many other countries, Nepal is going through a process of decentralization. The lead agency for the development and implementation of policy is the Department of Water Supply and Sewerage (DWSS), which falls under the Ministry of Physical Planning and Works (MPPW). Under the National Guidelines for Sanitation and Hygiene Promotion, 2005 and in line with policies relating to decentralization, responsibilities for sanitation provision are to be decentralized, with DWSS retaining an advisory and enabling role. DWSS is still in the process of determining what this role might mean in practice and has organized a series of regional workshops to explore future activities and responsibilities. It has defined the scope of the activities to be undertaken in its District and Regional offices, with a clear emphasis on water supply. References are made to sewerage, sewage treatment and cost recovery principles for sanitation schemes in small towns (by implication relating to sewerage and communal facilities) but there is no explicit mention of household sanitation.

Responsibility for implementation lies with Water User and Sanitation Committees (WUSCs). These are linked to Village Development Committees (VDCs), which in turn link upwards to the District Development Committees (DDCs), which are responsible for overall district-level planning. The whole decentralized DDC/VDC/WUSC structure falls under the Ministry of Local Development (MLD) and is supported technically by the District Technical Office (DTO). DTO staff are provided through the Department of Local Infrastructure Development and Agricultural Roads (DoLIDAR).

So, for rural and small town programmes at least, the policy and overall lead agency function is the responsibility of one ministry, while the day-to-day implementation of that policy is carried out by organizations falling under a second ministry. In practice, DWSS continues to be involved in the planning and implementation of schemes serving populations of over 1,000 through divisional and sub-divisional offices.

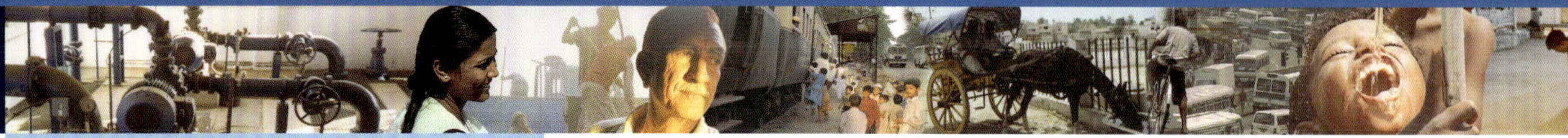

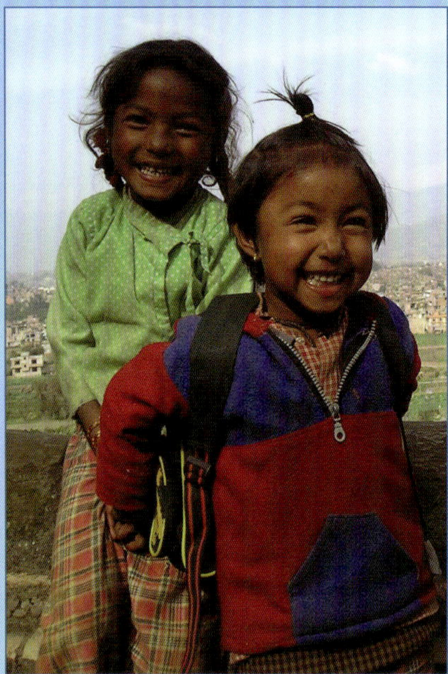

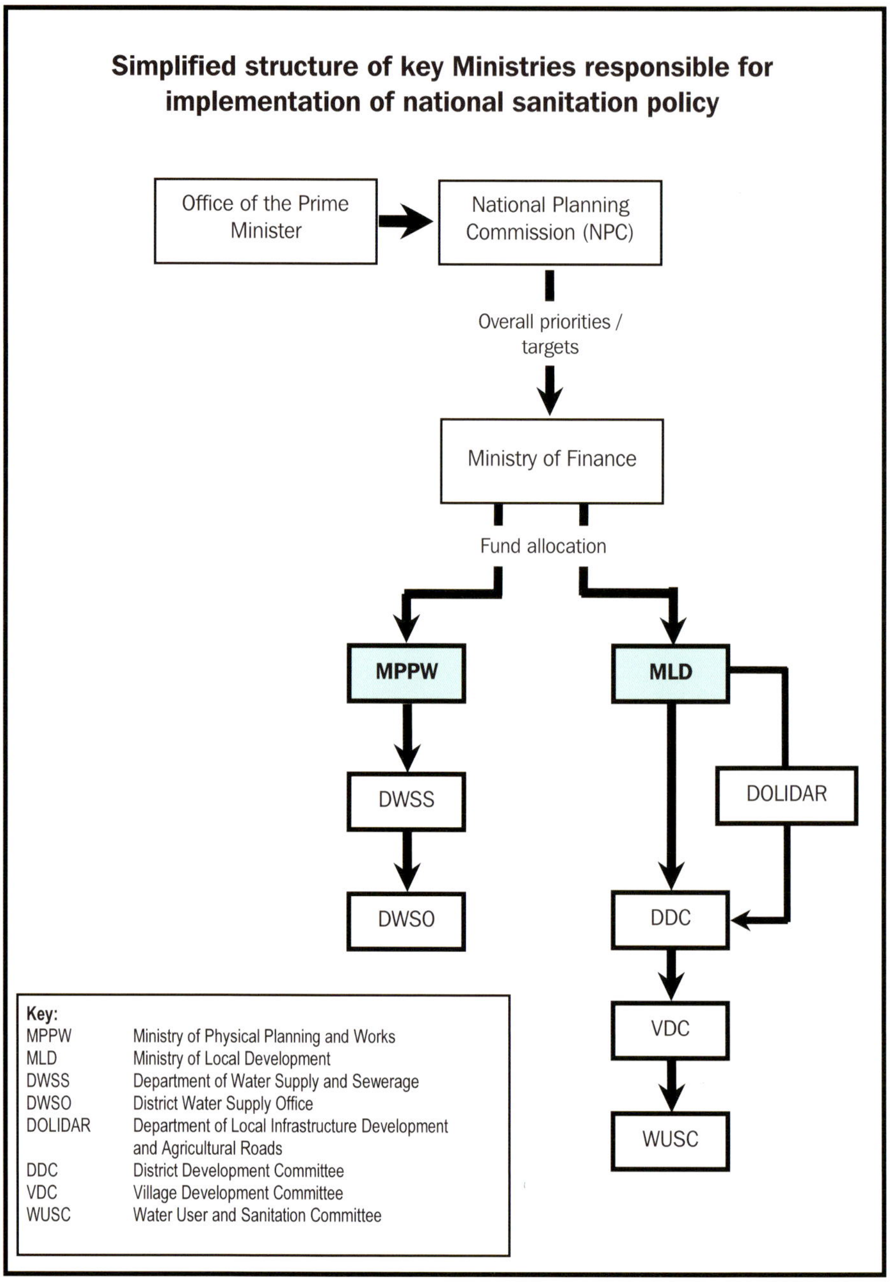

The result is a potential for misunderstanding and duplication of roles, as departments and district staff adjust to their new roles and responsibilities – some of which are not clearly identified in the policy documentation.

Efforts to resolve these issues have been hampered by the political situation, which has prevented local government bodies from functioning for the last three years.

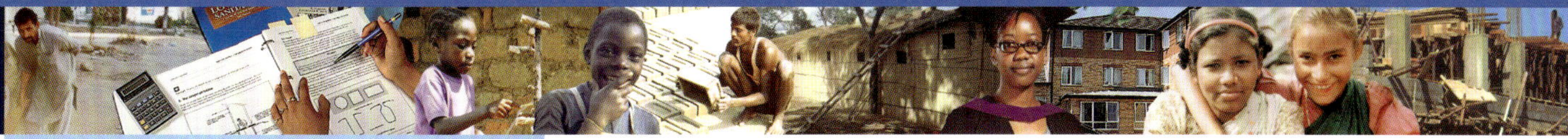

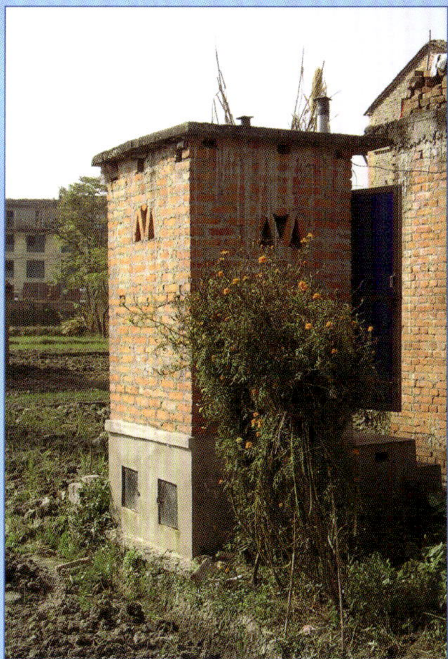

Resource gaps

Expenditure in the water and sanitation sector is currently dominated by water supply projects, in particular the Melamchi scheme, which is projected to require about 70% of the development budget available between 2000 and 2015. The shortfall in funds to support sanitation improvement and expansion is estimated to be about $6 million per year (WaterAid, 2004), about 54% of the level required to meet the MDG sanitation target. Given clear statements that there should be no subsidy for sanitation, much of this gap should theoretically be filled from people's own resources. The question then arises as to whether low-income households will be able and willing to build latrines without subsidy support and whether resources are available to promote improved sanitation.

There are also concerns regarding human resources as the sector adopts decentralized service provision. Local government bodies, with limited technical capacity struggle to fulfil the roles assigned to them by policy. Sanitation is not prioritized in locally generated plans and programmes, partly because household sanitation is not a shared 'public' responsibility. The DWSS's regional structure is remote from some districts and lack of coordination with ministries (notably health and education) means that other organizations with locally based human resources are not involved in promoting and supporting sanitation programmes. The result is that responsibility for promoting sanitation and supporting sanitation improvement efforts rests largely with NGOs.

Achievements and challenges

Focal point for co-ordination

Several key requirements of the 1994 National Sanitation Policy that were implemented have continued to influence developments in the sector. At the national level, the creation of a sanitation cell within DWSS provided a focal point for the coordination and development of sanitation-related efforts. Coordination arrangements stipulated in national sanitation policy have been put in place, including a National Steering Committee for Sanitation Action (NSCSA) and a Sector Stakeholders Group, covering both water supply and sanitation. District-level water and sanitation committees have been formed, although most meet infrequently. The National Sanitation Week, called for by the policy, has become an annual event.

Sanitation promotion workers

Unfortunately, some aspects of the 1994 policy remain unimplemented. The failure to appoint female sanitation supervisors in every district, with support staff including four female sanitation

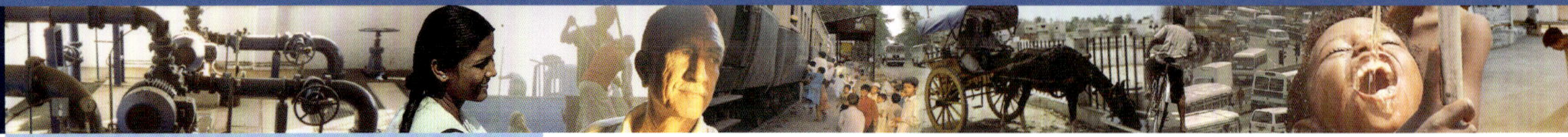

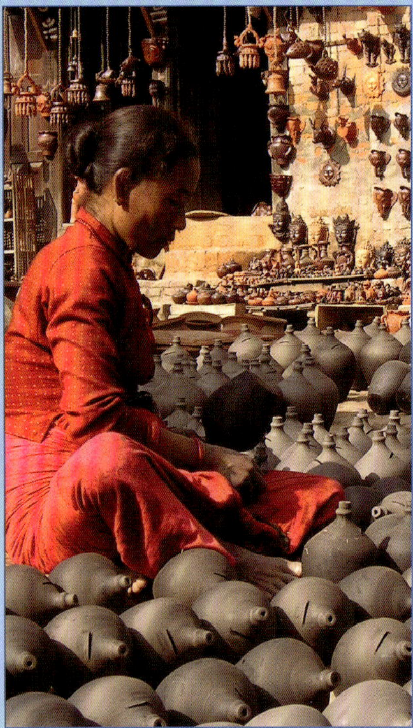

promotion workers, left a significant gap at the grassroots level in the key area of sanitation promotion. The 2005 guidelines omit this requirement, perhaps recognizing that it would be impossible to implement, although it does provide guidance on alternative approaches to sanitation promotion.

Coverage gap

After more than 10 years with a policy dedicated purely to sanitation, the gap between water supply and sanitation coverage remains at over 50% and is even greater in the Terai region. Planning at district level and below is crucial and the best way to facilitate improved sanitation coverage appears to be to implement stand-alone sanitation initiatives. This is unlikely to be a priority for the DTOs, while DWSS lacks the local presence required to support such initiatives.

Engaging other government actors

A key challenge is to engage departments and ministries other than DWSS and its parent ministry in policy implementation. While most recognize the existence of sanitation policy, they make limited use of it when planning their activities. There is a particular need to ensure that the National Planning Commission (NPC) and Ministry of Finance (MoF) actively support sanitation policy and ensure that it is reflected in poverty reduction papers and strategies.

Practice drives policy

While all NGOs within Nepal work within the basic decentralized arrangements required by policy in general, many recognize that their activities are situation rather than policy driven. Other aspects of policy, such as the role of women in sanitation promotion, the use of appropriate technology and the use of appropriate media channels to promote sanitation messages, are reflected in their activities. However, it appears that NGOs have emphasized these aspects because they are widely recognized as important, rather than because they are required to do so by policy.

Ways forward

Development of the National Guidelines for Sanitation and Hygiene Promotion, 2005 enables the sector to focus on improving implementation of policy. This will require ongoing review of the guidelines and action plans based on experience, although the eventual revision of the 1994 policy itself should also be considered.

Coverage data

There is currently considerable uncertainty about sanitation coverage figures. Measuring progress towards policy objectives requires efforts to develop an improved information-base on sanitation coverage and use.

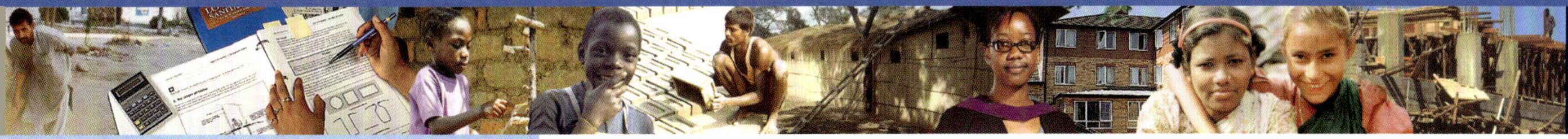

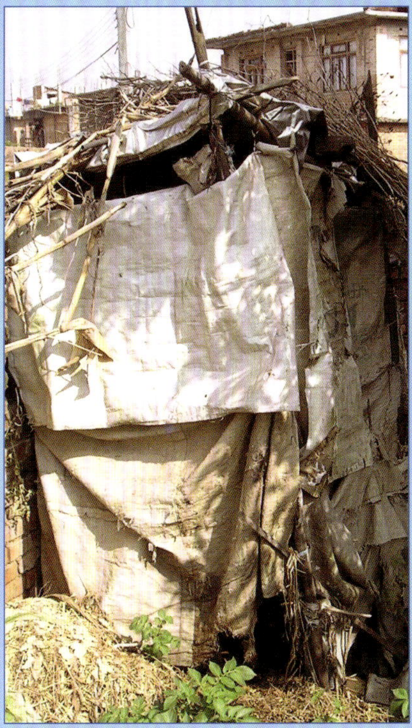

Targets

Efforts to implement policy should include a focus on improving sanitation coverage and use at district level. This will ensure that national targets are broken down into more realistic and therefore achievable local targets. It will also facilitate comparison between different districts and allow assessment of the factors that make some districts more successful than others. Focusing on the district level and below will also increase opportunities to assess the relationship between national policy requirements and practice in the field. This in turn will help to ensure that future revisions to policy are grounded in experience.

Promotion

Given the shortfall in funding, there is a strong case for an increased focus on promoting user awareness and creating informed demand for improved sanitation and hence increasing user willingness to contribute to the capital costs of improved facilities. Ministry of Health community level staff and Female Community Health Volunteers (FCHVs) could play an increased role in sanitation promotion. This will require closer liaison with the Ministry and, once the idea has been accepted in principle, technical and financial assistance to ensure that community-level health staff receive appropriate training and support.

Private sector

Opportunities for the private sector to work in partnership with government and the NGO community, supporting capacity gaps, should be further explored and optimized.

Co-ordination

There is a need to build on existing coordination arrangements, with the aim of widening government involvement in sanitation-related decision-making. Greater engagement with the National Planning Commission and Ministry of Finance is required to ensure that sanitation issues are adequately addressed in national poverty reduction programmes.

Footnotes

[1] The 25% figure is taken from the Tenth Five Year Plan. The 2000 national census suggested that 46% of the population had access to excreta disposal facilities but that half of these were 'temporary' facilities, a term used to denote unsatisfactory facilities.

[2] Urban coverage is estimated to be less than 70%, and rural coverage less than 20%.

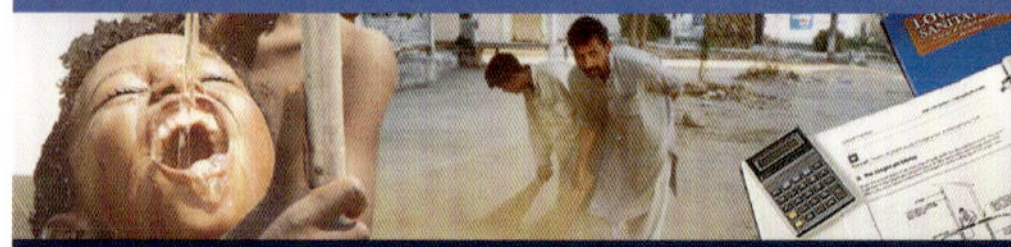

This Briefing Note presents an overview of key challenges and opportunities facing Nepal in the implementation of national sanitation policy.

It is based on the findings of research undertaken in 2003-2005, as part of a DFID-funded research project *Application of tools to support national sanitation policies (R8163)*.

Other research outputs include:

- Sanitation Policy: Why it is important and how to make it work – an overview guidance note.
- National sanitation policy in Ghana: a case for improved co-ordination? – a briefing note from Ghana.
- Comparing National Sanitation Policy Content – a note summarising and comparing the content of sanitation policies from 9 countries.

Key references

Elledge, M. F., Rosensweig, F. and Warner, D. B. (2002). *Guidelines for the assessment of national sanitation policies* (EHP strategic report no.2), Arlington, USA.

Tayler, K., Scott, R. and Shrestha, G. R. (2005). *Application of tools to support national sanitation policies: Assessment of Nepal's national sanitation policy*, WEDC, Loughborough University.

WaterAid, Nepal (2004). *The Water and Sanitation Millennium Development Targets in Nepal: What do they mean? What will they cost? Can Nepal meet them?*

This Briefing Note has been compiled by:
Kevin Tayler, independent consultant
Rebecca Scott, WEDC
Guna Raj Shrestha,
Development Network (P) Ltd, Nepal.

Photographs by Rebecca Scott

Published by WEDC, November 2005

This Briefing Note is part of a series covered by ISBN 1 84380 093 4 and was funded by the UK Department for International Development (DFID). The views expressed, however, are not necessarily those of DFID.

WEDC *People-centred solutions for sustainable development since 1971*

For more information contact:

Rebecca Scott or Andrew Cotton
Water, Engineering and Development Centre (WEDC)
Department of Civil and Building Engineering
Loughborough University
Leicestershire LE11 3TU UK

Telephone: +44 (0) 1509 222885
Fax: +44 (0) 1509 211079
Email: r.e.scott@Lboro.ac.uk
a.p.cotton@Lboro.ac.uk
Website: http://wedc.Lboro.ac.uk/projects/new_projects3.php?id=142

Briefing Note: Ghana

Assessing Sanitation Policy

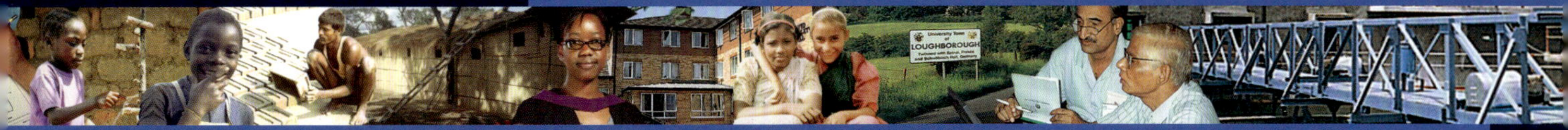

National Sanitation Policy in Ghana

A case for improved co-ordination?

WEDC

Summary

The best estimate of current sanitation coverage in Ghana is around 35% but there are significant regional variations with coverage in some regions being much lower. Despite the relatively low sanitation coverage, investment in sanitation, which is currently about $25 million per annum, is only about 25% of that in water supply.

Ghana has had a National Environmental Sanitation Policy since 1999. This takes a wide view of sanitation, covering food hygiene and solid waste and excreta disposal. Its decentralized approach reflects Ghana's commitment to developing decentralized forms of government. This Briefing Note has a narrower focus on excreta disposal.

The policy was developed by the Ministry of Local Government and Rural Development (MLGRD). It is a fairly concise document that sets out basic principles and objectives, identifies roles and responsibilities and also covers environmental management and protection, legislation and funding among others.

The Ministry of Works and Housing (MWH) has overall responsibility for water resources and supply and has developed policies and strategies that cover provision of 'water-related sanitation', which in essence means sewerage.

There is an urgent need for improved coordination between sector stakeholders. In particular, there is a need for shared policies and strategies that are owned by all the main stakeholder ministries and departments, clearly setting out the roles to be played by those ministries and departments.

Headline issues

- Sanitation coverage in Ghana remains fairly low, particularly in the Northern, Upper Eastern and Upper Western Regions. In each region, coverage does not exceed 20%.
- Diarrhoea accounts for around 25% of deaths of children under 5, highlighting an urgent need to raise awareness of the need for improved sanitation and hygiene.
- In theory, institutional responsibilities for sanitation are clear, with the Ministry of Local Government and Rural Development (MLGRD) having overall responsibility for formulating environmental sanitation policies. Water supply falls under the Ministry of Works and Housing (MWH).
- In practice, the MWH is involved in facilitating sanitation provision in rural areas and small towns, through its Community Water Supply and Sanitation Agency (CWSA).
- Ghana's National Environmental Sanitation Policy (ESP) dates from 1999. It sets out the roles of a number of ministries and institutions, but needs to be updated to include reference to the roles of MWH and CWSA. The policy mentions the role of the Ministry of Health in supporting hygiene education activities and contributing to regulation and standard setting for environmental sanitation services, but does not expand on what this role might entail.

There is a need to update policy to make good these deficiencies. While updating policy, the possibility of requiring that the various stakeholders working in the sector follow a sector-wide approach should be considered.

Loughborough University

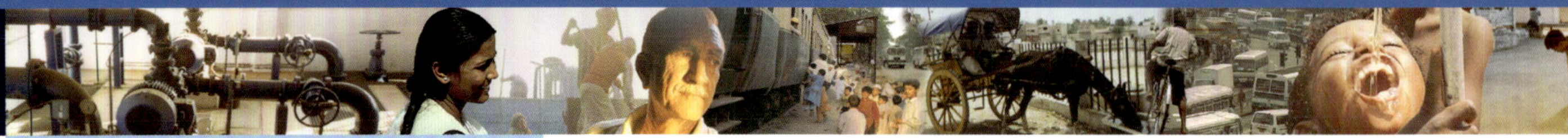

Background

Ghana's population in 2004 was about 20.6 million and growing at a rate of around 2.9% per annum. UN assessments suggest that the population will reach 26.4 million in 2010 and 33 million in 2020. About 42% of the population is urban and this figure is expected to grow to about 46% in 2015.

Infant and under five mortality rates had been steadily dropping until 1998 but then showed some increase in the period up to 2003, to 64 per thousand and 111 per thousand respectively. Deaths from diarrhoea account for around 25% of deaths in the under five age group, suggesting a need to create awareness of the importance of improved sanitation, provide improved facilities and promote improved hygiene.

There are variations between estimates of sanitation coverage. In its Strategic Investment Programme (SIP), the Community Water Supply and Sanitation Agency (CWSA) estimates current coverage figures of 31% for rural areas and 40% for urban areas, giving an overall national coverage of 35%. There are considerable regional variations, with coverage in the Upper Eastern Region only about 10% and that in the Northern and Upper Western Regions not exceeding 20%[1].

WHO figures indicate that annual investment in sanitation in Ghana over the period 1990 to 2000 was only about 25% of that in water supply[2]. The sanitation sector was heavily dependent on external funding, with over 90% of funds coming from donors and only $1.15 million per year funded from national sources. This heavy dependence on external funding has meant that the sector tends to be project driven. This is important because many projects are implemented through CWSA and focus heavily on water supply. Government's direct funding for water and sanitation has tended to decrease in recent years, but is likely to increase in the future as allocations are made from HIPC funds.

Ghana's sanitation policies and strategies

The National Environmental Sanitation Policy

Ghana's National Environmental Sanitation Policy (ESP) dates from 1999. It was prepared by the MLGRD in consultation with other stakeholders. The policy covers all aspects of environmental health, including excreta disposal and solid waste management. It sets out responsibilities for the various stakeholders, from individuals through community organizations to the MLGRD, Metropolitan, Municipal and District Assemblies (MMDAs), Ministries of Environment Science and Technology, Health and Education, educational institutions and the private sector.

In accordance with Ghana's overall commitment to decentralization, as reflected in the Constitution and various enabling acts, the policy assigns an enabling role to higher levels of government and the departments and agencies that fall under them. MMDAs are given direct responsibility for waste management, public health management, environmental monitoring, planning and monitoring. However, responsibility for developing appropriate environmental sanitation infrastructure, including domestic and communal toilets, rests with communities, which are directly responsible for planning, technology selection and implementation.

The policy makes no mention of the CWSA. The reasons for this are not clear, although one contributing factor may be the fact that CWSA was created while policy formulation was in progress. This is a serious omission, given the high reliance of sanitation programmes on external funding and the fact that much of the funding for rural and small towns is channelled through CWSA.

The National Water Policy

MWH has recently developed a National Water Policy, which consolidates three existing policy/strategy documents, prepared separately by CWSA, Ghana Water Company Ltd (GWCL) and the Water Resources Commission (WRC), into one policy. While the main focus of this document is on water supply, it does refer to sanitation.

It is probable that organizations such as CWSA, which fall under MWH, will look to this policy for guidance on sanitation-related matters rather than the more comprehensive Environmental Sanitation Policy. The result may be a tendency for sanitation to be marginalized.

Resource availability

Ghana has limited resources for sanitation development and this is reflected in the fact that over 90% of sanitation-related investment

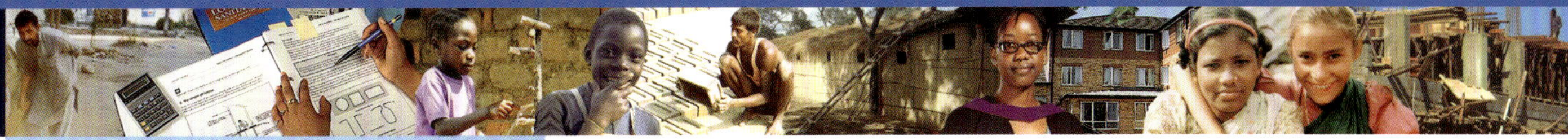

Institutional context

The 1992 constitution of Ghana created a vision of a decentralized system of public administration and governance. In accordance with this vision, successive local government acts have allocated significant powers to Metropolitan, Municipal and District Assemblies (MMDAs). The Local Government Act (Act 462) required the setting up of District Works Departments in District Assemblies (DAs)[3]. In practice these did not develop as intended. Projects are supported by District Water and Sanitation Teams (DWSTs), which are temporary project-level entities, created by CWSA as a stop-gap measure and staffed by people seconded from various departments within the DA. These lapse on the completion of projects and must then be revived to support subsequent projects.

DAs fall under the Ministry of Local Government and Rural Development (MLGRD), which has overall responsibility for formulating policies relating to environmental health and sanitation. The CWSA and its Regional Water Supply and Sanitation Teams (RWSTs) on the other hand, are part of the Ministry of Works and Housing (MWH), which is responsible for formulating polices relating to water supply and water resources.

The National Environmental Sanitation Policy Coordinating Council (NESPoCC) is responsible for coordinating activities relating to environmental sanitation. The Sanitation and Environmental Health Unit, housed within the MLGRD, acts as the secretariat to NESPoCC. It is also responsible for developing strategies for policy implementation and monitoring environmental sanitation aspects of Ghana's Poverty Reduction Strategy (GPRS) and MDG targets.

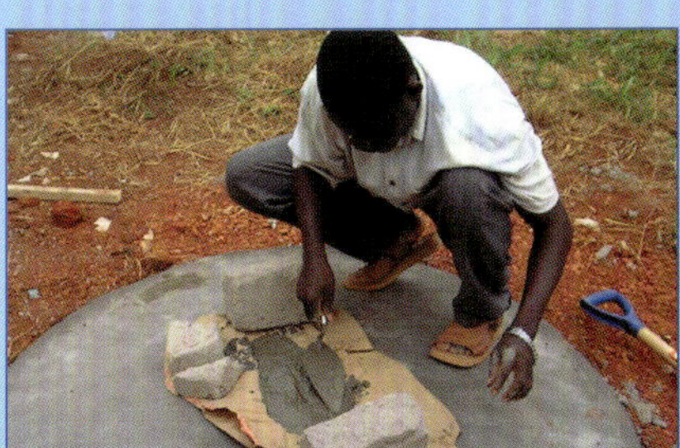

over the period 1990 – 2004 was externally funded (based on WHO figures). This suggests a need to ensure that international donors are aware of policy and work in accordance with it.

The available figures suggest that there will be a need for increased investment if the MDG sanitation target is to be met. An even greater increase in investment will be required to meet the higher target set out in CWSA's Strategic Investment Plan.

Achievements and challenges

- MLGRD is universally recognized as the lead ministry for sanitation policy development.
- The responsibility of MMDAs, which fall under MLGRD, for the implementation of development programmes, including sanitation, is recognized in the Constitution and Civil Service Law. The policy recommendations on decentralization are broadly being followed, although there are capacity issues at the local level.
- NESPoCC was formed in 2000, ceased to function in 2002, but has now been revived.
- The GPRS includes specific short term targets (2000-2005) for rural and urban sanitation, emphasizing the role of sanitation and water supply in achieving targets for reductions in infant and under-five mortality rates.
- A 'sanitation week' has been held annually as required by policy. The first day of the week, national Environmental Sanitation Day (ENSADA), is often accompanied by high level political participation and speeches.

Despite these achievements, challenges remain. The greatest of these is to develop policies and strategies that are accepted and followed by MLGRD and MWH, together with their subsidiary organizations. Each Ministry currently has its own priorities, programmes and procedures and makes little formal reference to the other.

Recommended actions

Specific recommended actions relating to policies, structures and strategic plans are:

- revise the environmental sanitation policy to reflect the role played by CWSA;
- seek convergence between the recommendations and requirements of the National Environmental Sanitation Policy and the National Water Policy;
- more clearly define the roles of the Ministries of Health and Environment in relation to sanitation and ensure that the Ministry of Health and its staff are actively involved in an integrated approach to sanitation promotion and provision; and

- reconcile the strategic planning and funding requirements of the Environmental Sanitation Policy and the National Community Water Supply and Sanitation Guidelines. The first requires that local authorities develop Strategic Sanitation Plans and calls for the creation of a District Environmental Sanitation Fund. The second requires District Water and Sanitation Plans and the creation of a District Water and Sanitation Fund.

Ways forward

Ghana clearly needs a revised environmental sanitation policy, which takes account of the roles played by all stakeholders, including the MWH and CWSA. In order to ensure that the policy is widely owned, particularly by the key ministries, the policy development process must be participatory. The team implementing the process should ideally be drawn from all key sector ministries, including Works and Housing, Finance, Environment and Health. MLGRD, as the lead sector ministry, should initiate and lead the process.

Donors can and should provide support for the development of the revised policy. As with national stakeholders, it will be important to consult them about the content of the policy. Conversely, it will be essential that donors then work within the overall framework provided by policy, rather than pursuing their own individual agendas. Ideally, they should do this through a shared Sector-wide Approach and this might be one point to be covered by policy.

Footnotes

[1] Annual Progress Report of the Ghana Poverty Reduction Strategy, 2003.

[2] WHO Global Water Supply and Sanitation Sector Assessment 2000 report, Africa Region, Part 1. http://www.who.int/water_sanitation_health/monitoring/globalassess/en/ (accessed Sept 2005).

[3] Municipal and Metropolitan Assemblies have different institutional arrangements and different names for their departments. The focus here is on the District Assemblies, with which CWSA mostly works.

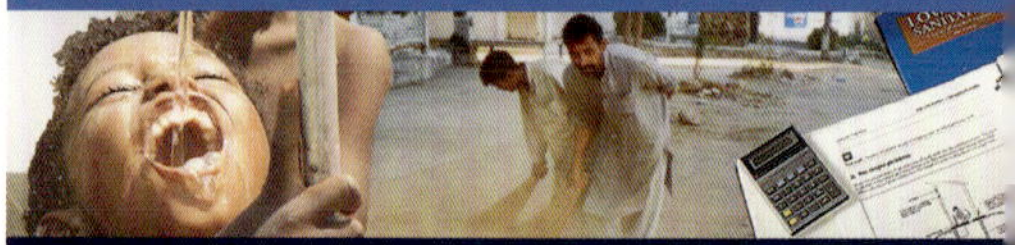

This Briefing Note presents an overview of key challenges and opportunities facing Ghana in the coordination and implementation of national sanitation policy.

It is based on the findings of research undertaken in 2003-2005, as part of a DFID-funded research project *Application of tools to support national sanitation policies (R8163).*

Other research outputs include:

- Sanitation Policy: Why it is important and how to make it work – an overview guidance note
- Implementing national sanitation policy in Nepal: challenges and opportunities – a briefing note from Nepal
- Comparing National Sanitation Policy Content – a note summarising and comparing the content of sanitation policies from 9 countries

Key references

Elledge, M. F., Rosensweig, F. and Warner, D. B. (2002). *Guidelines for the assessment of national sanitation policies* (EHP strategic report no.2), Arlington, USA.

This briefing note has been compiled by:
Kevin Tayler, independent consultant
Lukman Salifu, WaterAid, Ghana.

Photographs by Amaka E U Godfrey

Published by WEDC, November 2005

This Briefing Note is part of a series covered by ISBN 1 84380 093 4 and was funded by the UK Department for International Development (DFID). The views expressed, however, are not necessarily those of DFID.

WEDC *People-centred solutions for sustainable development since 1971*

For more information contact:

Rebecca Scott or Andrew Cotton
Water, Engineering and Development Centre (WEDC)
Department of Civil and Building Engineering
Loughborough University
Leicestershire LE11 3TU UK

Telephone: +44 (0) 1509 222885
Fax: +44 (0) 1509 211079
Email: r.e.scott@Lboro.ac.uk
a.p.cotton@Lboro.ac.uk
Website: http://wedc.Lboro.ac.uk/projects/new_projects3.php?=142